DISCLAIMER

The information presented is meant to help guide participants through practices that can help individuals become stronger and healthier through proper use. This information, however, does not promise any benefits when misused or misinterpreted. Please follow the guidelines as directed.

When participating in any exercise or training program there is a possibility of physical injury. If you engage in any movements, exercises or training programs, you agree to do so at your own risk. By voluntarily participating in these activities, you assume all risk of injury to yourself and agree to release and discharge Mathias Method, Ryan J. Mathias and all other affiliates of any responsibility if injury occurs. In addition, by following any of the suggested guidelines, protocols, templates, activities or any other information or advice given, you do so at your own risk. Do not begin any nutrition, health, exercise or training program without consulting with a Board Certified Medical Doctor and/or Registered Dietician first.

By utilizing this information presented you are stating that you agree to our Terms of Use which can be read in full on MathiasMethod.com/terms-use/.

ABOUT THE AUTHOR

Your STRENGTH JOURNEY Leader

Ryan J. Mathias

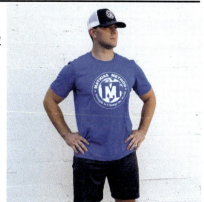

- **B.S. Degree in Exercise Science**
  - **Strength & Conditioning**
  - **Health & Fitness Concentrations**
- **Best Selling Author**
- **Competitive Powerlifter**
- **Teacher & Student of Strength**
- **World Changer**
- **Motivator**

Email: ryan@mathiasmethod.com

@StrengthJourneyLeader

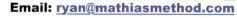

"I want to make the world stronger, and this is the only way I know how."

Hi, I am **Ryan Mathias,** Author of the this Best Selling Fitness Book and creator of the **MATHIAS METHOD STRENGTH SYSTEM**.

Some info you should know about me is, I am a competitive powerlifter with over **15 years of training experience**, all backed by a **Degree in Exercise Science** from California State University-Sacramento (CSUS). I am self-made with everything that I do, as I constantly pursue my dreams on a daily basis, with little to no guidance. I put my heart into everything I do and have the goal of helping as many people as I can along my Journey to Change The World!

Needless to say, I am **obsessed with STRENGTH!** I have always loved learning about and teaching people how to get stronger. Not only that, but I want it to be done properly to the best of my ability. I am always learning new things and improving my knowledge, and all that I learn I share with others, because no matter how strong I get, **we are all stronger together**. I hope you will choose to pursue your Strength Journey, and let me lead you along the way!

Also, I am a **3rd Degree Black Belt** with numerous martial art **Grand Champion** and **World Championship Titles** (2007-2010, 2013-2014, 2016). Much of my training, such as what you will read in the following, was developed not only to make me stronger, but also improve my athletic performance and keep my body healthy for my martial arts.

I developed the Mathias Method from my many successes and failures throughout my broad training experiences; in order to provide others with the best possible information that I can on how to get stronger! If you want to get updates about any new information that I learn, or want some training guidance, then go to MathiasMethod.com and start getting stronger today!

Email
ryan@mathiasmethod.com

with any **Questions**, **Comments**, **Stories** or **Reviews**!

I would love to hear from you!

OTHER BOOKS BY RYAN J. MATHIAS

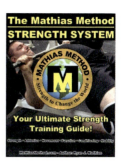

Mathias Method STRENGTH SYSTEM:

Your Ultimate Strength Training Guide!

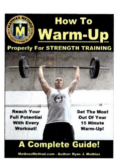

How To Warm-Up Properly For Strength Training:

A Complete Guide!

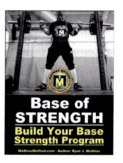

Base Of Strength:

Build Your Base Strength Program

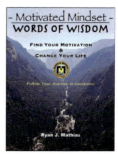

Motivated Mindset:

Find Your Motivation and Change Your Life!

DEDICATION

This information is dedicated to all those that believe in becoming stronger. Stronger through self-improvement and the pursuit of greater achievement. For those that always push for more and crave success. For those that don't let challenges stop them from doing what they set out to do. For all the dreamers out there, that keep their dreams alive! This information is dedicated to YOU, because YOU are the only one that can make a difference in your life. YOU are the only one that can Change YOUR World!

THANK YOU

Thank you to all those that read this information and believe in our mission to help Change The World through Strength. Thank you for standing with us.

SPECIAL THANK YOU TO:

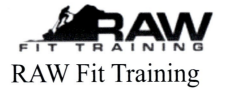

RAW Fit Training
3137 Swetzer Rd. Ste C
Loomis, CA 95650

PHONE #: (916) 367-6484
EMAIL: membership@rawfittraining.com

Thank you for allowing us to use your awesome facility to help make the world a stronger place!

The Daily 30

The Modified Daily 30

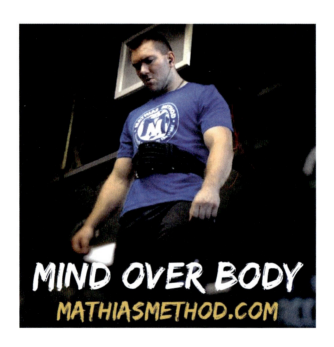

A NOTE FROM THE AUTHOR

Strength is the basis for all other Training Goals. I wish I would have known that, long ago, when I started my very own Strength Journey. As a short and large kid growing up with 3 brothers, **I always wanted to look better and get stronger.**

I started off doing some PTs my dad had my brothers and I do when we were little, then eventually grew into doing some weight training. All along the way, **I didn't have much guidance** on how to properly approach my goals. I would stop eating fat entirely as a young teen trying to lose body fat and would do a tremendous amount of push-ups, along with other various exercise, but **I was doing it all wrong**. Even when lifting weights in high school, I was not shown how to lift properly or create a successful program. **If only I would have been given a system to follow or a general plan to build upon I would have been set up for much greater success.**

Through all the struggles and failed attempts to make progress, **I learned many important lessons that helped me develop an incredible base of knowledge in which to build upon**.

After many years of slowly progressing, I continued to develop my training programs, and learn as much as could about making a strong body. I obtained my NASM (National Academy of Sports Medicine) **Personal Training Certificate**, and worked hard to get my **B.S. Degree in Exercise Science**, that together **helped me develop the Mathias Method Strength System**.

I had a long journey to get to where I am today, but I am glad I was able to suffer through, because I came out the other side so much stronger.

I started my Strength Journey by doing bodyweight workouts at home every day. I began doing 70 push-ups a day, then expanded into intense full body workouts. You can read more about that on my website, but overall the end result was, **I got really fit!**

However, my goal was to get strong, and I was doing it all wrong. Bodyweight movements can make you very strong, but the way I was doing them really wasn't benefiting me as much as it should have. **I was doing a bunch of random exercise variations with bad form** that taught me improper movement patterns and only made certain parts of my body strong.

What I should have been doing was focusing on **getting the most out of my workouts** by doing the most beneficial exercises for my body and learning proper movement patterns from them (especially as a growing teen)! **I should have been doing the Daily 30!**

With this knowledge in mind, I created this simple routine to help others avoid the downfalls that I had. **I want you to achieve your goals** without having all the struggles I had to go through. I made this book for those that want to do it all right. I made this book for YOU! Now, **let's start your Strength Journey…together!**

Strength To You,

Your STRENGTH JOURNEY Leader

Ryan J. Mathias

To read my complete Strength Journey, go to:

<u>MathiasMethod.com/My-Strength-Journey-Story/</u>

BODYWEIGHT FITNESS MADE EASY!

Throughout all of my training experience I have learned one important thing:

Fitness doesn't have to be hard!

Fitness and bodyweight strength training are not about being fancy, by doing advanced routines that are just too difficult for most people to perform reasonably. **It's about doing what works.**

Actually, it is usually the simple things that give the greatest results and overall benefit!

The Daily 30 is all about keeping things simple, fast and effective. This routine will teach you Basic Human Movements and hammer in the most effective exercises to help you get the most bang for your buck, while giving you the greatest results and preventing any risk of injury. You will learn how to move properly while building the strong, fit and healthy body you've always wanted!

This book is designed to give you a strong foundation using basic movements that can later be expanded upon as you do more exercises and add variation. You should always push yourself to do better, but never lose the foundation of movement you will develop with the Daily 30.

Note:

When exercising, how you do something is just as important as what you do!

It is much more beneficial to do basic exercises properly, than doing intense exercises poorly. Get good at the basics first, then you can expand upon them if you get bored, but always maintain your Foundation of Movement you will develop with the Daily 30. If the movement puts you in a compromised position, then just don't do it! Do what works, and do it well!

FITNESS IS A LIFESTYLE

Make fitness a part of your life every day!

One of the hardest things about fitness is sticking to it. It is so easy to neglect our bodies when we don't "feel like" doing what is necessary to maintain a healthy lifestyle. That is why the Daily 30 is daily. By doing this simple exercise routine daily you are so much more likely to stick to your fitness goals, and achieve them! You will always have this daily reminder that your health is important, and should not be neglected.

By choosing to improve your fitness you are choosing to live a healthier life for you, and those around you. You are choosing to make your health a priority so that you can be around for those that you care about most, and that care about you most.

For them, fitness needs to be a part of your everyday life. You need to remember to keep yourself hydrated, make healthy food choices, and exercise regularly. The more you neglect your body's health, the harder it will be to get back into your fit lifestyle. So choose to take just a few minutes every day, and improve your fitness. Make YOU a priority and you won't regret it!

A FOUNDATION OF MOVEMENT

Movement. It's the base behind any form of exercise. Movement alone will help cure and prevent most basic bodily pains and injuries. If we just move more, we will all be much healthier and have less pain. Not only that but if we move correctly we will increase our function to do anything and everything in life. We will be better at sports, get stronger, increase our mobility and so much more!

Movement Experts say that it takes 300-500 repetitions to learn a new movement pattern, and takes 3,000-5,000 repetitions to correct an improper movement pattern. That is why it's so important to move properly every day in order to constantly be improving the correct movement patterns and avoiding the wrong ones.

The Daily 30 is all about doing Basic Human Movements we all can do or should be able to do. These movements should be practiced daily for the most benefits and overall health improvement.

As humans, our bodies were designed to Squat, Push, and Pull. We were meant to do these exercises on a daily basis to keep our bodies strong and healthy. Over time, through the development of chairs, technology advancements, and overall living conditions, we lost a lot of the movement practice we were meant to do daily.

Today we see people with constant back problems, hip or knee pain, shoulder injuries and lack of overall fitness. This can all be fixed by simply taking the time to let our body move the way it is supposed to move every single day. Not only that, but we can use these movements to make a simple, yet highly effective bodyweight exercise routine that can literally be done by anyone of any age; anytime, anywhere! This workout will help anyone build a strong foundation of movement that will help you create the strong and healthy body you've always wanted!

This is the bodyweight workout we were all meant to do throughout our entire life to maintain a strong, healthy body, and it is so simple!

MOVEMENT BASED EXERCISE

All of the exercises in the Daily 30 are Basic Human Movements that our bodies already know how to do!

For example, the Paleo Squat is a great exercise to help decrease pain in your lower back, hips, knees, and ankles. This movement builds strength and muscle, while improving your flexibility!

We call it the Paleo Squat because it is a movement that has been ingrained into our anatomy since the Paleolithic Era. There were no chairs back then, and rocks are not always around to sit on, so humans would do a full depth squat, sitting on their ankles for rest. If you don't believe me, just watch an infant. When they go down to pick something up, what do they do? They squat down with their feet flat and sit on their ankles in a perfect squatting position! They look pretty comfortable too!

When they are laying down or crawling, what do they do? A push-up, and eventually push themselves up into a squatting position to stand! Then watch how they climb things. They don't jump onto things. They grab a hold of something with their little death gripping claws and pull themselves up, as we were designed to do!

You might notice that some African and Asian cultures maintain most of these movements because they have movement built into their culture. They still squat instead of using chairs, they do physical labor daily and are always being active with their bodies. It is those that are sedentary (without exercise) that have the worst movement patterns, overall health, and physical pains. Those that are constantly active tend to have much greater movement abilities, strength, health and the least amount of pain.

Again, we are born with these movement patterns of how to squat, push-up, and pull properly, but lose them over time through lack of practice as we grow. If we want to maintain or re-ingrain these movements into our body, we have to practice them every single day!

The more often we do them, the faster we will get them back and the better you will feel, guaranteed!

BASIC FOUNDATION EXERCISES

These basic foundation exercises are designed to build your full body strength, health, and fitness.

By going into the full depth Paleo Squat daily you will help to actively stretch out your muscles which in turn takes pressure off of your joints. The full depth position is especially great for spinal decompression, which is caused by bad posture, sitting and age. By simply performing this incredible exercise daily you can help to alleviate almost all of your muscle and joint pain!

Push-ups are a great way to improve our upper body strength! It not only works your arms, shoulders, and chest but your entire body from head to toe as you have to maintain a strong body position during the entire exercise. This promotes core strength during movement as you build up your body's stabilizers. Just remember, keep everything straight from head to toe! No mountain or valley hips (hips raised high or hips dropped low).

Now, most people cannot do a Pull-Up, so we made a modification to accommodate everyone by replacing the Pull-Up exercise with a Prone Cobra Exercise. The Prone Cobra is a Yoga Based Movement that works your entire posterior chain musculature helping to set our shoulders back in a better anatomical position while building core strength. This exercise works your entire back while stretching out our commonly tight chest and shoulder musculature, greatly improving our posture. If you have bad posture, this is a great way to correct it!

Every exercise in the Daily 30 can be tailored specifically to your current physical abilities. We even have modified versions for those with injuries, disabilities or physical limitations; and they will still make you feel GREAT!!!

WHAT IS THE DAILY 30?

The Daily 30 is a short and simple bodyweight exercise routine consisting of 3 exercises done for 10 repetitions each. These exercises are to be done at least once each and every day to teach your body to move safely using proper movement patterns. It **takes less than 2 minutes** to properly complete one round and will have an invaluable amount of benefits if done consistently over time.

WHAT ARE THE BENEFITS?

The main physical benefit of doing the Daily 30 properly on a regular basis is **increased neuromuscular proprioception**, also known as the "mind-muscle" connection. This teaches your body to move properly by stimulating the correct muscles while going through normal and compromised ranges of motion. By gaining this increased muscle activation your body will **better be able to protect itself from injury** caused by both improper repetitive motion and quick reflexive action, in everyday life.

<u>Other valuable benefits of the Daily 30 are:</u>

- **Increased Mobility**

- **Spinal Decompression**

- **Joint Stabilization**

- **Increased Body Control**

- **Improved Gastro-intestinal Health**

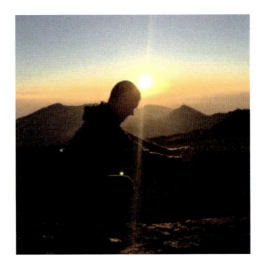

- **Improved Blood Flow Circulation**

- **Base Level Muscular Strength**

- **Joint Health**

- **Improved Posture and**

- **Builds Core Stabilization.**

16

WHO IS THE DAILY 30 FOR?

Everyone! The Daily 30 is made for anyone and everyone! Everyone can benefit from improving their functional movement patterns, increased neuromuscular proprioception, general strength and all the other benefits the Daily 30 provides.

Children can utilize it as a way to develop their body's strength and movement patterns from a young age.

Teens can use it to help maintain their strength and mobility as their bodies grow.

Adults can use it to stay active throughout the day while on break at work to increase body function or as an hourly active stretching routine to rejuvenate between long sitting sessions.

Seniors can use it as their daily activity to feel better, decrease pain and get in some beneficial exercise.

Anyone can use it as a way to train at home (when done for multiple rounds), or while on the road traveling.

Strength athletes and all others can, and should, use it as part of their warm-up before a training session, which will reinforce proper lifting technique while preparing their body's for the training they are about to do.

It can even be used as a form of rehabilitation from injured or dysfunctioning muscle groups. The Daily 30 is simple and can be used by anyone to help improve their health and get stronger. So go get started today, and remember to have your friends and family join in!

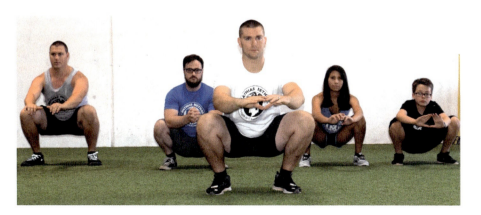

WHAT IS THE PURPOSE?

The main purpose of the Daily 30 is to **keep you dedicated to your health and fitness goals through the self-discipline** it takes to do it each and every day.

There will be many days that you don't "feel like" doing the Daily 30, the same as you don't always "feel like" doing everything else that is needed for you to be successful in life. By doing the Daily 30 each and every day, **no matter how you feel**, you will remind yourself to always **stay focused on your goals** and take steps towards them everyday.

Just by doing one simple act every day, you can **start to change your world**, because every small act done towards a specific goal will lead you to success. So take action and start changing your world every day, no matter how you feel. Stay focused, maintain self-discipline, and Change Your World!

WHEN'S THE BEST TIME TO DO THE DAILY 30?

1.)   Part of Your Workout Warm-Up

The best time to do the Daily 30 is as part of your Warm-Up routine before any workout. No matter what you do for a workout, you should incorporate a Warm-Up routine of some kind to gain the most benefit from your training session. The Daily 30 should be incorporated because it helps take your body through full ranges of motion, strengthening proper movement patterns, while improving mobility and improving muscular function, all while increasing your muscular temperature. All of this together will allow you to train more optimally and safely.

We recommend you do the Daily 30 1-5 times before every training session as part of your warm-up. Also be ensure to include other training specific warm-up exercises as needed.

2.)   Morning

Though immediately upon waking, while your body is still preparing for activity, is not the most optimal time for exercise, about an hour after waking up is a great time for you to do the Daily 30. At this time your body has had enough time to prepare for your daily activity and you are ready for action. By starting your day off with the Daily 30, you re-enforce strong movement patterns that will help you move properly throughout the rest of the day. Every time you go to sit down, or move your arms, or are just standing up, your body will remember to be in a better position so that you have less pain throughout the day. By doing the Daily 30 every morning you will simply teach it to move properly throughout the day with little thought put into it.

We recommend you do the Daily 30 1-3 times every morning, an hour after waking.

3.)   All Day Every Day

Anywhere, anytime! The main purpose of the Daily 30, along with all the physical benefits, is that it teaches consistency. It teaches you to always be focused on improving yourself and working towards your own goals, wether that be to get stronger, be healthy, or anything you have. Use the Daily 30 as a reminder to always push for progress in life every day. So not matter how late is is, how tired you are, how much you do not want too, always DO YOUR DAILY 30!

No one is going to change your world for you. YOU have to be the change and it starts with doing things that will benefit you, wether you feel like doing them or not. No go change your world!

The Daily 30

Exercise 1

PALEO SQUAT

10 Repetitions

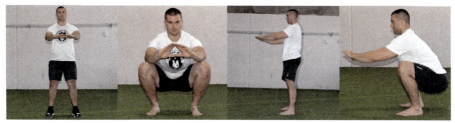

Stand with your feet shoulder width apart and toes straight or turned out slightly. Clench your feet into the ground as if they were eagle claws (creating a slight arch in your foot) and externally rotate (twist) your knees out during the entire movement, while bracing your glutes and core.

Begin the motion by pushing your hips back 3 inches and leaning forward slightly, then open your hips and descending straight down into a full depth squat, bending your knees and hips at the same time. (Note: Only go as deep as you can while keeping your heels down) Pause at the bottom position for two-seconds before reversing the motion to stand erect.

Make sure that your knee moves in line with your toes during the entire range of motion! Don't let them cave in, as this is a dangerous knee position. Also, focus on having your hips go back and down, then forward and up.

Do a total of 10 repetitions.

Benefits

Some physical benefits of the Paleo Squat are increased gastrointestinal health, spinal decompression, improved muscular function, proper joint movement, and hip, knee and ankle flexibility.

> Tip: If you lack the flexibility to go into a full depth squat comfortably then hold onto a solid object for stability and stay in the bottom position for extensive time (5-10 minutes) in order to gain flexibility.

Purpose

Teach proper squatting mechanics, improve blood flow, improve mobility, alleviate muscle and joint pain, and increases overall health and fitness.

Prime Movers - Most Active Muscles

Quadriceps (Legs), Glutes (Hips), Hamstrings (Legs)

Exercise 2

PUSH-UP

10 Repetitions

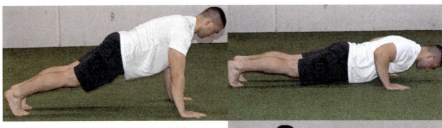

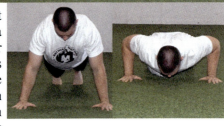

Place your hands shoulder width apart and feet together with your body in a straight line from head to heels. Your fingers should be spread as wide as possible, with your glutes and core braced. While keeping your hands in place, create an external rotation torque during the entire motion, the same as you did with your feet during the Paleo Squat.

Descend until your body is barely hovering over the floor, pause and then press back to the top position.

Do a total of 10 repetitions.

If you cannot do a push-up on a flat surface, adjust by placing your hands on an elevated surface. As you increase strength, lower the elevation each week until you can do a full push-up. Keep all the same protocols and do not do push-ups from your knees, because this teaches a bracing fault and will decrease your strength potential. See the *Modified Daily 30* (pg. 28).

Benefits

The push-up increases upper body strength, builds core stability and teaches proper movement patterns for the shoulder and elbow joint.

> Tips: Flex your glutes to help brace your torso to your legs and keep your head neutral.

Purpose

Teaches proper arm and shoulder pressing mechanics and builds upper body strength.

Prime Movers - Most Active Muscles

Triceps (Arms), Anterior Deltoids (Shoulders), Pectoralis Major (Chest)

Exercise 3

PRONE COBRA

10 Repetitions

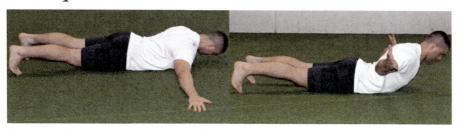

Lie face down on the ground with your arms out to your sides making a T-shape with your body. During the entire motion keep your fingers spread wide, glutes activated and balls of your feet kicked into the ground; raising your knees.

With a neutral head position, begin by raising your torso as high as possible while externally rotating your palms upward (thumbs pointing up). Think of pulling your shoulder blades back down towards your glutes and thumbs together behind you. Hold the top position for two seconds and then slowly return to the start position. Do not fully relax to the floor and repeat.

Do a total of 10 repetitions.

Benefits

The prone cobra builds the strength and mobility to hold proper posture.

> Tips: Keep tension on your legs and glutes for stability. Brace your core by pressing your navel out against the floor.

Purpose

Teach thoracic extension and shoulder external rotation while building postural strength.

Prime Movers - Most Active Muscles

Erector Spinae muscles (Back), Rear Deltoids (Shoulders), Trapezius (Back), Rotary Cuff Complex (Shoulders)

DO YOU WANT TO ADD MORE?

Go to MathiasMethod.com/all-training-exercises/ to view all of our Exercise How To's which can be added to your daily routine for even more benefits!

<u>Notes:</u>

Date you first started doing the Daily 30:

_____

How many Push-Ups can you do in a row:

Day 1?_____   Day 30?_____

How do you feel after doing the Daily 30:

On Day 1?

On Day 30?

What are your goals?

THE DAILY 30 WORKOUT!

The Daily 30 is designed as a fast, simple and effective bodyweight exercise routine that teaches you to move properly while increasing your mobility and strength, among other things. However, doing the Daily 30 only a few times randomly throughout the day will not make you very fit, trim, or build a ton of muscle. **To use the Daily 30 as a fitness routine you have to do it quickly, numerous times, and treat it as a workout circuit**.

I recommend that you **set a timer for 10, 15, or 20+ minutes and see how many rounds of the Daily 30 you can complete** within that time frame. That turns it into a real butt kicking workout pretty quick, and you will feel the effects afterwards! By doing this, strength may be a limiting factor, so you can do the easier modified version of some exercises if needed.

Another option for your workout circuit is to **do each exercise for a certain amount of time,** and keep switching between each exercise until the time is up, or you've completed a set amount of rounds. For example, **do each individual exercise continuously for 30-60 seconds,** then switch to the next and repeat. Just remember to push yourself and only rest when needed. Good Luck!

It is not necessary, but you can also add on any other exercises to your daily routine for even greater benefits!

Go to MathiasMethod.com/all-training-exercises/ **to view all of our Exercise How To's which can be added to your daily routine for even more benefits!**

Think you can handle it?

How many days in a row have you done the Daily 30? _____

How many times can you do the Daily 30 in…

10 min.?_____   20 min.?_____   30 min.?_____

How many reps can you do in 60 seconds?

Paleo Squat_____   Push-up_____   Prone Cobra_____

<u>Memories:</u>

(Put your adventurous pictures here!)

WHERE CAN YOU DAILY 30?

We want to see your Daily 30 pics! Take the best pictures you can and send them to us at

ryan@mathiasmethod.com

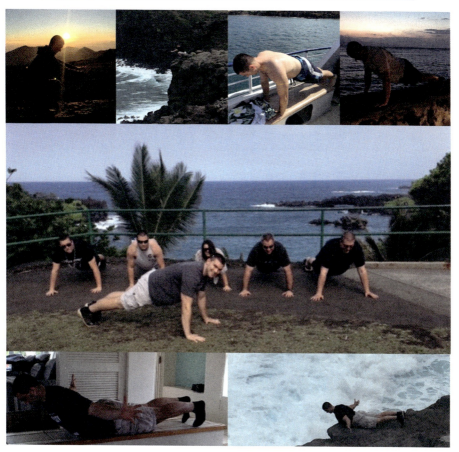

<u>You can Daily 30 anywhere!</u>

Even on Vacation in Hawaii (Maui)!

We want to see your adventurous pictures!

The Modified

Daily 30

These are easier variations of the Daily 30 exercises for individuals that cannot perform the standard Daily 30 exercises.

Exercise 1

ASSISTED PALEO SQUAT

10 Repetitions

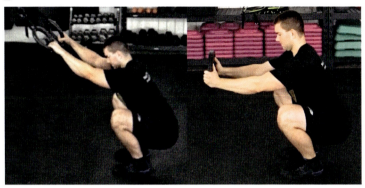

Hold onto a stable object, or hold a counter balance weight in front of you, for balance. Stand with your feet shoulder width apart and toes straight or turned out slightly. Clench your feet into the ground as if they were eagle claws (creating a slight arch in your foot) and externally rotate (twist) your knees out during the entire movement, while bracing your glutes and core.

Begin the motion by pushing your hips back 3 inches and leaning forward slightly, then open your hips and descending straight down into a full depth squat, bending your knees and hips at the same time. (Note: Only go as deep as you can while keeping your heels down) Pause at the bottom position for two-seconds before reversing the motion to stand erect.

Make sure that your knee moves in line with your toes during the entire range of motion! Don't let them cave in, as this is a dangerous knee position. Also, focus on having your hips go back and down, then forward and up.

Do a total of 10 repetitions.

Benefits

Some physical benefits of the Paleo Squat are increased gastrointestinal health, spinal decompression, improved muscular function, proper joint movement, and hip, knee and ankle flexibility.

Purpose

Teach proper squatting mechanics, improve blood flow, improve mobility, alleviate muscle and joint pain, and increases overall health and fitness.

Prime Movers - Most Active Muscles

Quadriceps (Legs), Glutes (Hips), Hamstrings (Legs)

Exercise 2

DECLINE PUSH-UP

10 Repetitions

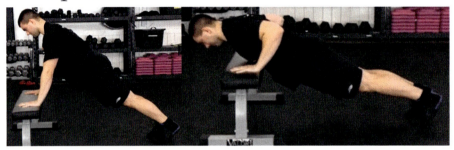

Place your hands shoulder width apart on a flat surface, hip height or lower, and set your feet together with your body in a straight line from head to heels. Your fingers should be spread as wide as possible, with your glutes and core braced. While keeping your hands in place, create an external rotation torque during the entire motion, the same as you did with your feet during the Paleo Squat.

Descend until your body is barely hovering over the flat surface, pause and then press back to the top position.

Do a total of 10 repetitions.

Benefits

The push-up increases upper body strength, builds core stability and teaches proper movement patterns for the shoulder and elbow joint.

> Tips: Flex your glutes to help brace your torso to your legs and keep your head neutral.

Purpose

Teaches proper arm and shoulder pressing mechanics and builds upper body strength.

Prime Movers - Most Active Muscles

Triceps (Arms), Anterior Deltoids (Shoulders), Pectoralis Major (Chest)

Exercise 3

STANDING PRONE COBRA

10 Repetitions

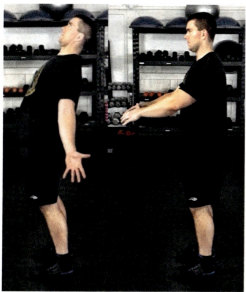

Stand erect with your hands touching together in front of you. During the entire motion keep your fingers spread wide, glutes activated and feet clenched into the ground with an external rotation torque. Brace your core by tightening your stomach along with all the muscles surrounding your abdomen.

With a neutral head position, begin by externally rotating your palms outward as you open your chest and lean back. Think of pulling your shoulder blades back and down towards your glutes and thumbs together behind you.

Only lean back as far as you can maintain balance. Hold that position for two seconds and then slowly return to the start.

Do a total of 10 repetitions.

Benefits

The prone cobra builds the strength and mobility to hold proper posture.

> Tips: Keep tension on your legs and glutes for stability. Brace your core by pressing your navel out against the floor.

Purpose

Teach thoracic extension and shoulder external rotation while building postural strength.

Prime Movers - Most Active Muscles

Erector Spinae muscles (Back), Rear Deltoids (Shoulders), Trapezius (Back), Rotary Cuff Complex (Shoulders)

THE DAILY 30 CHALLENGE

I challenge you to improve your strength, health and fitness by doing the Daily 30 at least once everyday, for 30 days!

Take photos on your first day, doing each of the motions. Then take photos from the same angle on the 30th day to see how much you have improved! See and feel how your body has changed in just one month!

Finally, write about your experience and submit it along with all of your before and after photos to ryan@mathiasmethod.com, and you could be featured on **MathiasMethod.com**!

Are you Self-Disciplined enough?

Let's find out...

Be sure to check out

MathiasMethod.com

Your FREE Online Strength, Health & Fitness Resource!

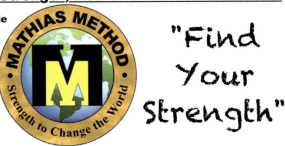

- Strength Training Guide
- Self-Assessment Guide
- Exercise Descriptions
- Informative Articles
- Nutrition Principles
- FREE Programs
- FREE Advice
- Motivation
- Videos

"Find Your Strength"

Learn How to Get Stronger No Matter Where You Start From!
Guidance From Beginner To Elite

PLEASE LEAVE A REVIEW!

Good Reviews are like gold to Authors, yet most Readers that like a book never write a review!

Not only does it warm our hearts knowing that our hard work, (and yes writing is very hard to do, as most books take months if not years to write, and just as long to publish and start selling.) has helped others, but it helps spread the word to others so that they too can benefit from it.

Just the same, bad reviews, and even average reviews, can hurt how a book is presented to others. I take pride in saying that everything in this book was written straight from the heart, and I hope to have presented the best quality of wisdom that I could, for you to learn from. Still, **I want to do better!**

I want you to give an honest opinion of this book, but if there is anything that you feel was missing, you misunderstood, or that I can help you with, list your suggestions in your review and please **contact me directly** so that I can continue to lend my services to you. So when you are done, please let me know what you think!

Go to **MathiasMethod.com** for FREE training programs and strength training information.

Do you know someone that would benefit from this book?

Share it with them!

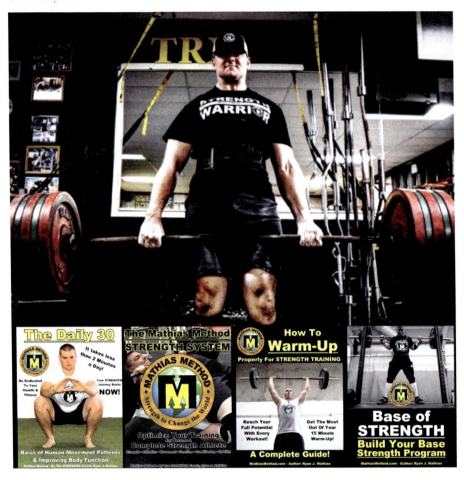

Learn more about me and check out all my other books on my Amazon Author Page!

Amazon.com/Author/RyanMathias

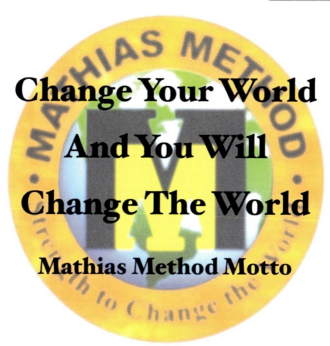

Change The World

We are on a mission to Change The World! We know that **we cannot do this alone** so we encourage YOU and all others to join us on this mission. **Join the Mathias Method Army** and make a difference today!

Being part of the Mathias Method Army means that **you believe in changing your world, in order to help others change theirs**. By continually pushing yourself to become better and get stronger everyday, you are helping to motivate others to do the same. **Others around you will come to you looking for encouragement** to start making changes in their lives alongside you. **This is your opportunity to make a difference** in their lives by helping them get stronger mentally and physically. **Keep a positive mindset**, no matter the challenges you face, and **always push to be better than yesterday**. Set goals, stick to them, and celebrate even small accomplishments. Changing the world will not be easy, but believe in yourself and you can do it.

Improve your life, and you can help to change the world!

Join us on **MathiasMethod.com** today!

Become a part of the

Mathias Method Army today!

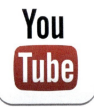
SUBSCRIBE to our YouTube

Mathias Method

| Exercise How To's | Informative Videos | Competition Videos | Motivational Videos |

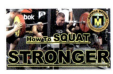 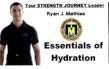 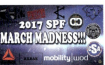 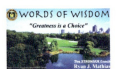

Follow Us On:

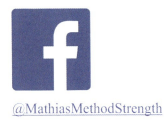 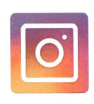 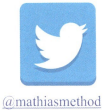

@MathiasMethodStrength   @mathiasmethod   @mathiasmethod

Check Out Our
STRENGTH APPAREL

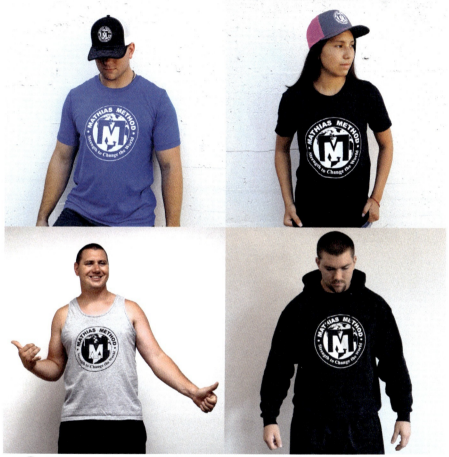

StrengthWorld.Store

Use Discount Code "Daily30Everyday" for 30% OFF
as a gift for reading this eBook!

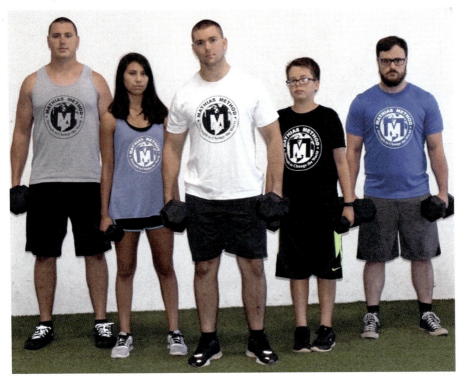

Stand Strong
and
Change Your World!

Made in the USA
Middletown, DE
25 July 2019